# DIY Sunburn Recipes:

## 40 Homemade Natural Remedies To Heal Sunburns

Table of content

## Introduction

Sunburn is a common type of burn during summer season. When a person suffers from this kind of burn, then the skin turns red and itchy. In severe cases, it can also cause blisters and swelling. Therefore, a cure to these kinds of burns is quintessential to avoid any damage to the skin. In order to get an efficient treatment to this burn, we have suggested some home-made recipes that will calm the sufferer's craving for itching. Moreover, since these recipes involve all organic products, they will be extremely useful as well as harmless.

The book includes forty recipes to treat this burn. Firstly, home-made remedies for sunburn are discussed in general. Secondly, special recipes for face burn are discussed. Thirdly, sunburn treatments created by using Aloe Vera and coconut oil are discussed. Fourthly, techniques to calm down the heat and itching faced by an individual during sunburn are explained in detail and along with some remedial suggestions. Lastly, the recipes to cure sunburn with things that are common in all households are given.

Thus, this book contains in itself forty home-made recipes to cure sunburn. This book possesses great importance because all of the recipes discussed here are efficacious and easy to make. Moreover, these recipes are safe as well as inexpensive as compared to the chemical cures suggested by pharmaceutical companies.

## Chapter 1 – Homemade Remedies for Sunburn

In order to fulfill the required amount of Vitamin D, sunlight is extremely important. However, if the exposure is excessive, then it might result in sunburn. An interesting fact about sunburn is that one must not have to take a sunbath to have it; it can happen even if your body is exposed to ultraviolet radiations from the sun. As your skin is a sensitive organ, therefore you must take extra care of it. Another important fact regarding sunburn is, the symptoms of this burn might take some hours to become evident. It might happen after an exposure to sun on for a small time, but on the hottest day.

The impact of ultraviolet radiations on a human DNA is similar to that of a nuclear radiation. As a result, the immune system of the body becomes active and kills the damaged cells to avoid harm to the rest of the body. This burn might make your skin red. This redness and the itching are just the price which your body pays to get rid of those damaged cells. Moreover, the production of melanin is blocked to avoid any movement of the damaging rays. This blockage results in darkening the body, usually known as tanning. After your body is tanned, the sun exposure is not capable to cause any further burn.

**Prevention:**

Despite everything, it is better to avoid sunburn in the first place. The damage caused to the DNA might have an impact on the aging of your skin. Thus your skin becomes old before its actual time. Moreover, this can also result in skin cancer. However, if we have suffered from the awful burning, then we must start looking out for ways that can be used to soothe the pain caused by the burn. A lot of homemade recipes are available that can be used to cure it. Interestingly, all of these recipes use natural ingredients which are commonly used in routine life.

It is a known fact that people with lighter skin are usually prone to skin issues like sunburn. However, other than this the intensity of sunlight as well as the duration for which the skin was exposed to the sun also matter a lot. It is, therefore, essential to choose the appropriate remedy. Despite being safe, the homemade recipes might not always work. If the condition is severe, it is always better to consult a doctor.

**Recipes for mild sunburns:**

In case you are suffering from sunburn which is partially red and touching it gives you a heat sensation, the sunburn is mild. At this point of time, you need to wash your body with a face wash. Rub it gently on your body; this will soothe your body. Further, some of the other things which might help you are as follows:

1. **Milk:**

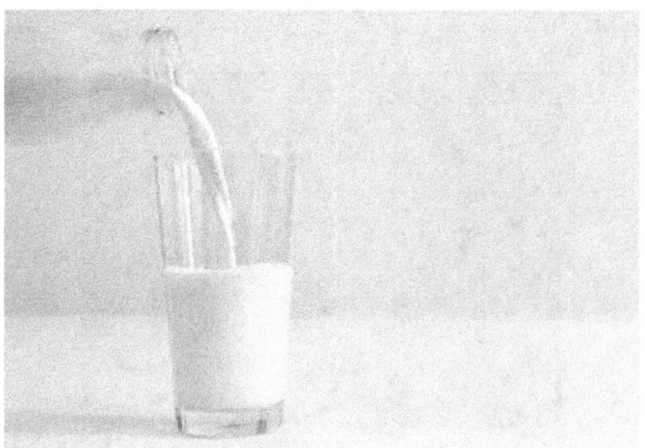

Milk is a common household item. Therefore, it is the best option to soothe your mild sunburns. You can apply milk on your burns if you are not allergic to the content of milk. This will provide apparent results after you rub it for some time.

Before applying milk on your body, wash your body with simple water and let it dry. After you have washed all of the affected parts, apply milk on the parts using a soft sponge or a pad. However, if you do not like the smell of milk then you can add your favorite oil in it to remove the smell. The addition of oil is totally up to you. After you have applied the milk, let it dry for some time on your skin. As a result, slightly thin layer of milk will be created. Now wash the skin after some hours.

Repeat this process several times to get steady results. Additionally, you can use skimmed milk as well. This will help you in avoiding all the fat on your skin that is caused because of the usual milk.

## 2. Cornstarch:

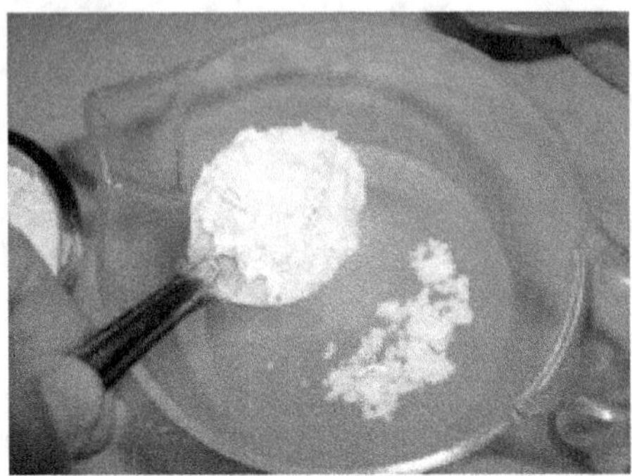

Cornstarch is a common cure used for all types of skin rashes. One can utilize cornstarch in numerous forms i.e., paste or powdered form. In order to apply cornstarch, use your fingers and apply the easily separable paste to the burnt area. Moreover, apply cornstarch, in powder form, on a damp skin to avoid chafing while you are asleep.

## 3. Tomatoes:

Tomatoes are a rich source of lycopene, which possess an antioxidant power. As sunburn is caused in a result of damaged tissues, these damaged tissues are accompanied with free radicals. These free radicals are highly reactive; therefore, anti-oxidizing agent is required to nullify their impact.

In order to cure mild sunburns, you either use tomatoes in the form of juices or you can apply it directly on your burn with a soft pad. However, drinking tomato juices are highly recommended to kill the reactive radicals that are capable of causing further skin damage.

*Recipes for serious sunburns:*
Some of the recipes to cure serious sunburns are as follows:

### 4. Coconut oil and milk:

Coconut milk is a high source of lauric acid, possessing efficacious antimicrobial agent. It is used to improve the cell growth. Moreover, it repairs the damaged cells. Coconut oil is a widespread remedy for sunburn in tropical areas, since it is free in those areas.

In order to use it, grate fresh coconuts and out them in mild warm water for some time. After that grind the mixture and pass it through a sieve.

Moreover, in order to cure the burnt part of the body, this oil directly can be applied directly.

### 5. Oatmeal and lavender oils:

Another remedy for sunburn is to take a bath and oatmeal and lavender oil in the water. In aromatherapy, oils are considered as a soothing cure for skin problems.

In order to apply it, grind the oatmeal and add some drops of lavender oil in it. Prepare a hot water bath by adding this mixture to the hot water in a tub. Take bath for a few minutes to avoid skin dryness.

*Recipe for extremely severe sunburns:*
### 6. Honey:

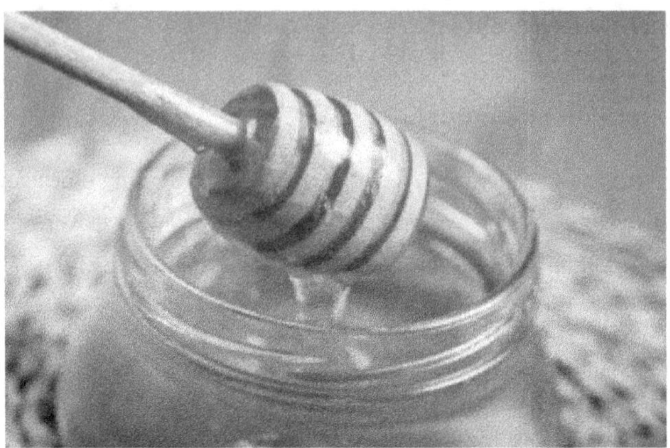

Honey is a readily available sunburn ingredient. Not only it possesses antibacterial characteristics, but also, it is hydrophilic. It is useful to cure the skin blisters and suck the liquid out of them. The fluid, present inside the blisters, is useful in healing the damaged tissues.

By applying honey, the blisters will infect the other tissues. In order to increase its sticking time, add some ground oatmeal to it.

## Chapter 2 – Sunburn Recipes for Face

While there are many organic ways to cure sunburn, your face is a very sensitive part of the body. Therefore, the remedies for face must be harmless than others. Some of the common sunburn recipes for face are discussed below in the coming text. By applying these on your face, you will not only cure your sunburn, but also, your skin will glow.

7. **Potato paste:**

Potatoes are considered as extremely good pain relievers. Therefore, you use them to eradicate skin irritations. Moreover, potatoes paste soothes the burns and scratches. Some of the people use potato juice to cure the burns while others use the slices. Both of them have efficient results.

In order to apply it to the burn, wash and grate the potatoes. Make a liquid out of them by grinding these grated potatoes. With the help of cotton balls, apply the liquid on your sunburn and let it stay for a while. Moreover, you can simplify put the slices on your face.

8. **Mint and tea:**

Mint has a natural quality to soothe everything which it touches. Therefore, it is also used to cure and calm your face sunburns. Green tea is also helpful in relieving pain since they contain tannic acid as well as theobromine.

In order to use it, add fresh mint and some tea bags to a little boiling water. Let it boil for some time and then strain. After chilling it for some time, you can apply the mixture on your burns. Moreover, green tea can be replaced by black tea.

## 9. Apple cider vinegar:

Vinegar is a household ingredient which is used to cure burns. Interestingly, apple cider vinegar is one of the best ingredients used to cure sunburn.

In order to use it, first take a bath with fresh water. Put this liquid in a spray bottle. Use this spray bottle to apply the liquid on your burns Let it dry for some time.

## 10.Witch hazel:

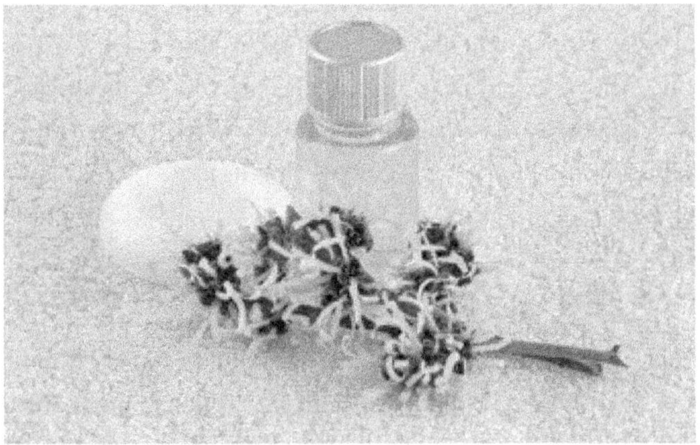

Use dry witch hazel plants in order to cure your sunburn. This herb is found in a liquid form in the markets to facilitate the user. Add the required amount of witch hazel in a jar, soak cotton balls in it and apply to the burnt places. Repeat this process after some time to get better results.

11. **Plain yogurt:**

Yogurt contains probiotics as well as enzymes that are used to improve the skin condition. In order to cure the sunburn, take some plain yogurt with probiotics, and apply the cool yogurt on the burnt parts to relieve pain. Once you feel relieved, wash it with fresh water. However, wash your hands thoroughly before applying the yogurt.

12. **Cucumber:**

Cucumber is used as an antioxidant to heal the burnt skin. Moreover, its analgesic properties are a source of relief from the pain caused by the burn. It can be used in numerous ways; however, each of those ways is responsible in the eradication of pain, swelling and redness.

In order to apply it, slice the cucumber and place it on your burns. Flip the sides when they are heated. However, to get better results, blend the cucumbers and make a paste. Apply this paste on the burns. Moreover, to increase the impact, add aloe gel or baking soda in the paste.

## Chapter 3 – Aloe Vera and Coconut Oil Sunburn Treatment

Aloe vera is an extremely useful ingredient, which cures sunburn along with many other problems. Some of the benefits of aloe vera are as follows:

- It contains numerous useful elements. Following are some of the elements found in aloe vera:

    i.      Zinc.

    ii.     Minerals.

    iii.    Tannins.

    iv.     Calcium.

    v.      Magnesium.

    vi.     Sodium.

    vii.    Copper.

    viii.   Manganese.

    ix.     Vitamins.

    x.      Amino acids.

    xi.     Germanium.

    xii.    Selenium.

    xiii.   Potassium.

- Aloe vera contains glycoproteins, which are used to cure body pain. Moreover, they eradicate inflammation as well.

- Moreover, the ability of aloe vera to repair damaged skin and tissues is derived from the polysaccharides present in it. Moreover, these polysaccharides further help in the formation of new cells.

- Aloe vera is very important since it contains capability to avoid heat sensation in the skin. Moreover, they stop the swelling of skin and body parts.

- The lidocaines of aloe vera are very important as well. They serve as an anesthetic. This results in removal of heat sensation as well as pain.

- Another amazing feature of aloe vera is the aloectin B. This element helps an individual to heal. As it has the ability to strengthen the immune system and consequently, speed up the healing of damaged parts.

- While considering the importance of aloe vera in burnt skins, it has an ability to create a protective layer around your skin. This layer, thus, prevent any further damage to the burnt part. Moreover, it stops the flux of moisture to heal the burnt area.

- An efficient quality of aloe vera is that it has no oils, therefore any irritation or oiliness does not occur on the skin. Therefore, pores are not clogged on the skin.

- Aloe vera also holds importance because it has an ability to fight bacteria. Bacterium is an infection causing microbe that must be cured.

- The ability of aloe vera gel to go deep into the layer helps in pain reduction and avoids the chance of swelling.

When a person is exposed to UVA and UVB rays for a long time, then he/she can experience blisters and redness because of sunburn. These burns can lead to numerous severe skin issues that can cause wrinkles, scars and dark spots. Therefore, it is essential to cure these burns. The best choice for sunburn cure is aloe vera. The coming text expounds upon the use of aloe and the way it can work.

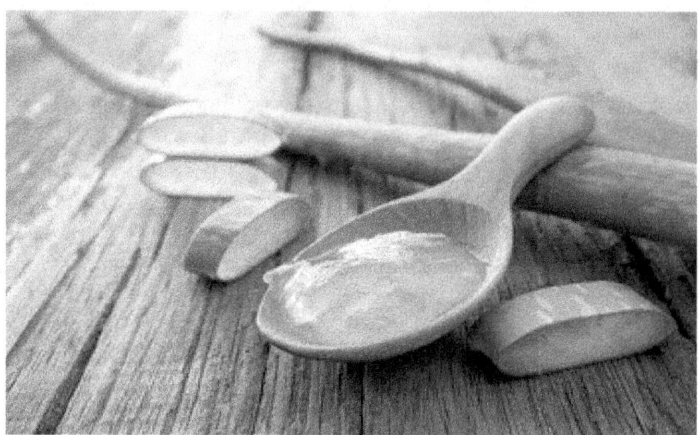

Aloe vera is very efficacious when used alone and even when used with other organic ingredients. This results in skin repair and lightening as well. Do try all of the methods explained below to get better results, depending upon your skin type. To get the optimum results, use fresh gel and juices which are used to make numerous pastes. However, you must make sure that the kind of aloe vera you use is harmless for your skin. In case you get severe burns, consult a doctor.

### 13. Natural gel:

To begin, cut a leaf of an aloe vera plant and take the gel out of it using your hand. Apply it using your hand or a soft pad. Let it stay on your burn until it is dried. Afterwards, rinse using cold water. Moreover, repeat this application after some time to get better results.

### 14. Cucumber:

To begin, take out aloe vera gel with the help of your hand. Then, take a cucumber wash and peel it. Afterwards, blend them together in a mixture to create a paste. Now put this mixture on your body parts. Afterwards, dry it for some time. This will eradicate the redness and soothe the scratching.

## 15. Herbs, cornstarch and aloe vera:

In order to cure sunburns, some of the herbs are very efficacious. Moreover, when these herbs are combined together with aloe vera and baking soda, their impact becomes great. To create this mixture, mix aloe vera gel, water and an efficient herb, in this case, witch hazel, in a ratio of 1:2:1. After mixing them, set them aside for about four hours. Add a few teaspoons of cornstarch in them. Keep in the refrigerator for one day in an airtight container. In addition, you can also add mint leaves in the mixture before keeping it in the refrigerator.

In order to get better result, apply this time 3-4 times a day.

## 16. Aloe vera and yogurt:

To create a sunburn cream using yogurt and aloe vera, extract gel from aloe vera leaves. Grate a cucumber and grind them together in a blender. Afterwards, put some yogurt in it and grind them together.  After the mixture is ready, put it on your burnt parts and leave them for thirty minutes. After the paste is dry, peel it off using fresh water. After you have washed the burnt areas, dry the skin and clean it. To increase the pace of recovery, apply the paste daily.

## 17. Aloe vera lotion:

In order to make this customized lotion, following ingredients are required:

- Aloe vera gel.

- Emulsifying wax.

- Vitamin C powder.

- Carrots.

- Cucumber.

- Beeswax.

- Sesame oil.

To begin, peel cucumber and carrots and grate them. Afterwards, cook these two in sesame oil for about half an hour. While cooking, care must be taken that the residue does not stick to the cooking jar. After cooking for thirty minutes, strain the vegetables and add both waxes and combine them together. Later add aloe vera along with Vitamin C powder and combine the mixture until it turns creamy. When it becomes smooth, remove it from heat and place it in the refrigerator. Use it 3 days a day to get better results. Store the remaining lotion in refrigerator. This lotion can be used within 2 months of its creation.

## 18.Aloe vera ice:

This is another efficient technique used in order to relieve the pain caused because of the sunburn. If you desire you create an aloe vera ice, take the gel out of aloe leaves, place them in special jars or trays and then put them in refrigerators. Once they are frozen, rub them on the burns to feel relieved.

Coconut oil is extremely useful kind oil. It is not only beneficial for skin cares, but also, for hair cares and other health care products. Moreover, it is not only common in tropical regions, but also, in UK and USA. This oil has continued to surprise people with its uses and benefits. It has numerous methods to cure sunburns, but only a few are discussed here. The coming recipes expound upon the use of coconut oil to treat sunburns.

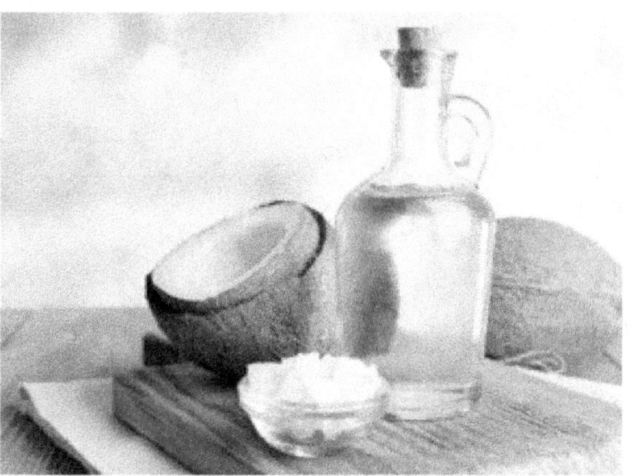

### 19. Coconut oil:

When you cannot find any other way to cure your sunburn, hop on the coconut oil. Coconut oil is a great source of nourishment for your skin. In order to get even better results, add some Vitamin E oil in a cup filled with coconut oil.

### 20. Coconut oil to cure lips:

Sunburn has a negative impact on your lips as well; therefore, a special remedy is added in here to cure these burns. In order to cure your lips, gently massage virgin coconut oil on your lips. This will improve the condition of your lips. Leave it on your lips for quite some time. Regularly repeat the procedure to get better results.

## Chapter 4 – Recipes to Cool the Sunburn

Sunburn can be very irritating as well as dangerous for the skin. Once a person gets sunburnt, he/she feels the desire to keep on scratching the burn. When a person scratches the burn, he makes it worse. When you scratch, the scars of those blisters become permanent. Therefore, one must not scratch the burnt areas. When a person suffers from sunburn, there arises a need to scratch them to relieve the pain. However, scratching does not help. In order to relieve the pain, use following recipes that will cool the sunburn:

### 21. Mint:

Mint is one of the most efficient ingredients to calm your desire to scratch. The mint leaves provide a cold sensation to your body. Therefore, use the mint to quench the desire to scratch. In order to apply it, either make a tea or add a few drops of mint oil in mildly warm water. Let the mixture cool for some time and then apply on the burnt areas.

### 22. Aloe vera:

Along with many other uses, aloe is also used to calm the sunburnt body parts. Aloe vera is capable of relieving the pain because it has lidocaine, this anesthetic helps in soothing the burn. Moreover, aloe vera is extremely good at peeling the skin.

### 23. Vitamin E:

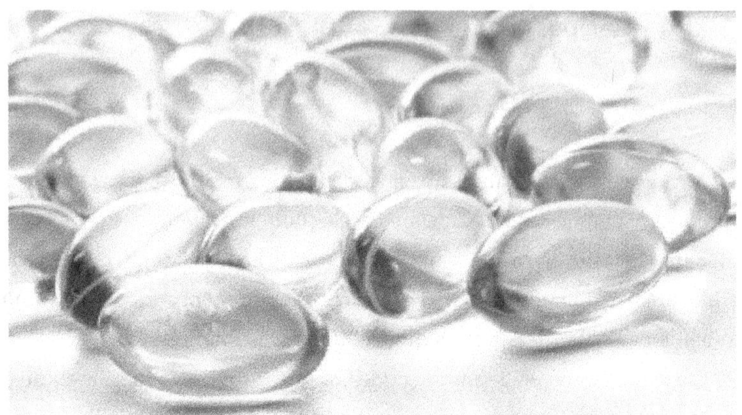

Vitamin E can be used to eradicate the sunburn and itching because of its antioxidant nature. The ingredient can be used in multiple ways. Some of the ways are as follows:

- Vitamin E can be taken in the form of supplements.

- Vitamin E is available in oil form. Therefore, you can rub it on the burnt part and get relieved.

- Vitamin E is also available in powdered form. Thus, allowing you to sprinkle it on the burnt parts of your body.

## 24.Black tea:

Black tea can also be used to cool the sunburnt skin of your body. To begin, boil the tea and cool it. Then, apply this cold tea on your burnt body parts. The presence of tannic acid in the tea helps in sucking the heat from your body and further balancing the pH of your body and skin. In order to enhance the cooling effect, add some mint leaves in the tea. This will calm down your desire to scratch the burnt parts.

**25.Chilled cucumbers:**

Cucumbers are used as natural healers for sunburns. Applying chilled cucumber paste on the burnt parts will help you in cooling the burnt parts.

## Chapter 5 – 15 Treatment of Sunburn with Things Always in hand

Treatment for sunburn can be expansive; however, you can cure the burn using the things which are commonly found in households. By utilizing these things, you will not only save your money, but also, these remedies are harmless. Some of the recipes that can be used to treat sunburn and are made up of the things that are usually found in homes are given below:

**26. Application of lettuce:**

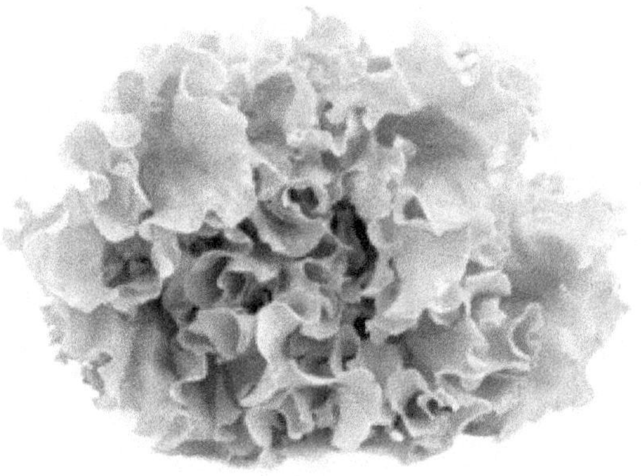

In order to cure sunburn, lettuce can be used. To begin, boil its leaves and let it cool down for some time. Afterwards, strain the leaves. In order to apply dip soft pads or cotton balls into the boiled water. And then softly rub it to the burnt parts. This will help you treat the sunburn.

### 27.Use ice:

Another method to treat sunburn is by using ice. When you got sunburn, you always desire to put something cold on your burnt parts. Therefore, take an ice pack and wrap a cloth around it. The pack is wrapped to make a mild impact.

### 28.Apricots:

Apricot is another household ingredient used to cure sunburn. In order to apply it on the burnt parts, first wash the apricot and peel it. Afterwards, create a paste of apricots. Then, apply this paste on your body.

### 29.Lotion:

Lotions are present in usually all of the houses. Therefore, to cure mild sunburn, you can use lotions. However, try to use those lotions which have least chemicals in it. Try to apply the lotion with antioxidants and probiotics. These will help you in curing your damaged tissues.

### 30.Egg white:

Egg whites are also efficacious in treating the sunburns. To begin, you need to separate the egg yolk and egg white. After that, whisk the egg white till it becomes smooth. Afterwards, apply this whisked egg white on the burnt parts of your body. This will result in sudden pain relief. Now leave it for some time and let it dry. Then, wash it off with fresh water.

### 31.Shaving cream:

Shaving creams contain methanol which clearly doubles the healing rate. Therefore, it can be used to cure the burns and scratching.

## 32. Strawberries:

Strawberries are a rich source of tannic acid; therefore, they can be used to cure sunburns. In order to cure your burns, grab some strawberries and make a paste of them. Afterwards, apply this paste on your burnt body parts for some time and then wash it using fresh water. The application of strawberries is useful because it will suck the sting out of the sunburn.

## 33. Use washcloth:

In order to cure the sunburn, dip a washcloth in cold water. After dipping it apply directly to the burnt areas. Whenever, you desire to cool your burns, apply the similar washcloth on your burns. This will provide a cold sensation to your body. Moreover, you can add certain ingredients in the water to increase the soothing effect. Some of the ingredients you can add in fresh water are as follows:

- Essential oils.

- Baking soda.

- Lavender oils.

- Ground oatmeal.

## 34. Tropical anesthetic:

Tropical anesthetics contain lidocaine, which is quintessential to cure sunburn. Moreover, lidocaine does not cause allergic reaction. Before using these tropical anesthetics on your burnt parts, try to use them on a small patch of your skin. Tropical anesthetics are found both as sprays and creams. However, sprays are comparatively more effective because they are easier to apply. Instead of spraying separately on all the burns, spray it at one place of a body part and spray it on the other burnt areas of the same spot.

### 35. Vegetable juices:

Tomatoes have an acidic nature; therefore, their juice can be used to cure sunburn. More importantly, it does not hurt when you apply tomato juice on your burn. On the contrary, it calms down your desire to scratch. Moreover, if repeatedly used, this can be the ultimate cure of your burn. Interestingly, the sun protection factor of tomato has close proximity to a lower level SPF.

### 36. Vinegar:

Vinegar can be used to treat the sunburn. Vinegar can do its work by simply applying mild quantity of vinegar on the burn. Vinegar can either be applied using the soft pads or spray bottles. The method adopted to apply vinegar is simple, yet it is quite efficacious. Moreover, vinegar reduces the chances of blisters. This is a huge application, since blisters are usually formed during sunburn.

### 37. Skim milk:

Another household ingredient for killing the burns is the use of skim milk. Add water into the skim milk and some essential oils if you desire. Afterwards, mix them together and create a fluid to apply on the burn. Once you have applied the liquid on your burns, you will feel calmness. This is because of the efficient ability of skim milk to soothe your pain.

## 38. Noxzema facial cleanser:

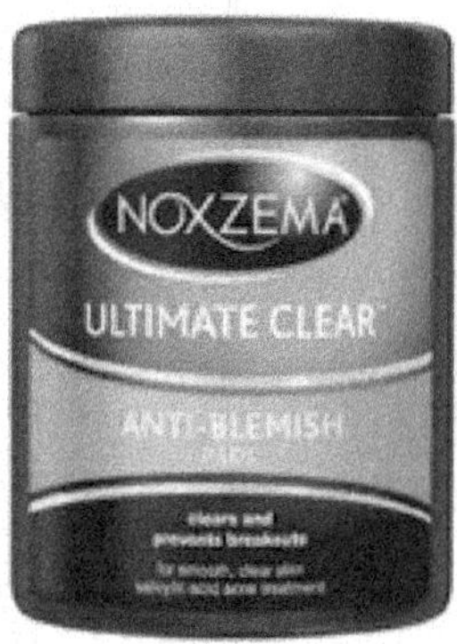

Another weird, but efficient thing to cure sunburn is Noxzema facial cleanser. This has a positive impact in curing facial sunburns. Therefore, it is utilized by a lot of men and women.

## 39. Avocado:

Avocado is usually used by people to cure their sunburns. Its use is very simple yet effective. To begin, peel off the avocado and mash it. Make a paste of the avocados. Afterwards, apply the paste on the burnt parts of your body. This will help you in eradicating the pain you have been suffering from sunburns. Moreover, this will lighten your skin; thus removing the chances of dark spots, scars or bags.

## 40.Petroleum jelly:

Petroleum jelly is a very common thing in all households. This can be used to treat your lip sunburns. Therefore, whenever your lips are burnt, try putting some petroleum jelly on them. This will increase the moisture in your lips and the content of this jelly will help you recover. Moreover, the damaged tissues or skin will be peeled off if you use this jelly. Thus, it is a very simple cure for sunburns.

# Conclusion

To conclude, sunburn is an awful burn caused because of excessive sun exposure. As a result of it, the skin of sufferer is severely damaged. Itching and blisters are also caused during the hideous burn. Therefore, it is essential to cure the disease and in order to cure it; numerous pharmaceutical companies as well as cosmetic brands are focusing on creating some of the creams. However, these creams contain numerous chemicals which can be harmful to the skin.

Thus, it is necessary to use such creams and treatments which are not harmful. Therefore, this book fulfills the need of this hour by providing forty such homemade recipes which can cure sunburn. These recipes are not only organic, but also, harmless. Moreover, these homemade recipes can be cheaper as compared to the expensive creams created by some of the famous brands.

The book is divided into five chapters. These chapters provide detailed recipes to cure sunburn. To begin with, the first chapter incorporates a general overview of homemade remedies for sunburn along with some of the recipes. Furthermore, the second chapter is comprised of sunburn curing recipes that can be used on the face. Moreover, the third chapter is about Aloe Vera and Coconut oil sunburn treatments. In addition, the fourth chapter provides the recipes that can be used to eradicate itching and pain caused because of the sunburn. In the end, the last chapter includes fifteen such treatments which can be created using common household things. Therefore, this book serves as a guide to home-made sunburn treatment.